This Notebook Belongs to:

____

Made in the USA
Las Vegas, NV
30 April 2021

22213423R10069